COUNTRY DOCTOR

PERSONAL EXPERIENCES & OBSERVATIONS IN PRIMARY CARE, 1960s & BEYOND

HAROLD CONLEY MD

ACKNOWLEDGEMENT

Special thanks to my son, Patrick, for his much-appreciated and essential help in the editing, formatting, design and guidance through the technology maze necessary to bring my vision, this book, to fruition.

FOREWORD

On many occasions in the past, while working at the Dells Clinic in Wisconsin Dells, Wisconsin, I was told by many of the personnel that I worked with that I should write a book about my experiences. At the time, I never gave it much thought, but since I have been retired, and have more time on my hands, I decided to describe, in general, the nature of primary care in the 1960s, and in the years thereafter, and how things differed so much from today.

For background information, first I will document some details of my education that led up to my MD degree and then some details of my postgraduate training before I went into general practice in Wisconsin Dells, Wisconsin. Then I will describe, in generalities, the nature of general practice in a rural area, such as Wisconsin Dells, in those days. Then, more specifically, I'll categorize the broad range of problems that I encountered in day to day practice over the years. Finally, I'll describe in some detail, a few situations that presented to me, for which I was responsible for providing care. Of course, this is hardly an exhaustive list, as there were countless others, of similar nature, during those years, but they will give the reader a sense of the variety and nature of what a primary care physician was faced with, and responsible for in those days. At least that was my experience.

As to my early life, I grew up during the "Great Depression" in a very rural area in southern Illinois. My parents had very little in terms of material assets and their ability to assist me financially in my education was extremely limited. Consequently, during my college education journey, I worked at a great variety of part-time jobs. The Pharmacy degree I obtained, I came to realize, was to become invaluable, if not an essential factor, in allowing me to pursue my MD degree.

SOME BACKGROUND INFORMATION REGARDING MY FORMAL EDUCATION, MEDICAL TRAINING AND EXPERIENCE

1947-1949
Attended Eastern Illinois State College in Charleston, Illinois
Major - Pre Pharmacy

1949-1952
Attended Butler University College of Pharmacy in Indianapolis, Indiana
Degree - BS in Pharmacy
Became Registered Pharmacist in Indiana by passing State of Indiana Pharmacy Board Exam

1952-1953
Attended University of Illinois Graduate School in Chicago, Illinois
Major - Pharmacology - (Drug Research)
Obtained Registered Pharmacy License in Illinois by reciprocity
Worked as Night Pharmacist at University of Illinois Research Hospital.

This involved being on call every other night, and the night on call, filling all the various hospital ward order baskets for drug supplies, and being on call for any other pharmacy needs that arose in the hospital during the night.
Hospital was 400 - 500 beds
Compensation was room in Hospital, shared with the other night Pharmacist, board (hospital cafeteria), laundry and $50 per month.

September 1953 - September 1955
US Army with service in Korea and Japan

1955 - 1959
Attended University of Illinois College of Medicine in Chicago, Illinois
Degree - Doctor of Medicine (MD)

During all these four years, I again worked as Night Pharmacist at University of Illinois Research Hospital. Again, this involved being on call every other night and the night on call, filling all the various hospital ward order baskets and taking Pharmacy calls during the night. Compensation was room in Hospital, shared with the other night Pharmacist, board (hospital cafeteria), laundry and $50 per month.

June 1959 - October 1960
Rotating Internship at Cook County Hospital in Chicago, Illinois

1960
Became licensed Physician and Surgeon in State of Illinois by exam

1960
Became licensed Physician and Surgeon in State of Wisconsin by Reciprocity (meeting with State Board of Medical Examiners and passing their exam)

1974
Became a Diplomate of the American Board of Family Medicine by passing their Board exam Continued to be certified by Board examination every six years

November 1960 - December 2002
Practiced Medicine at Dells Clinic, Wisconsin Dells, Wisconsin

Internship
Cook County Hospital
Chicago, Illinois
1959-1960

After my graduation, and receiving my MD degree from the University of Illinois College of Medicine in Chicago, I applied for Internship at Cook County Hospital, that was located just across the street from the University of Illinois College of Medicine. This location was just three miles west of the Chicago "Loop" in downtown Chicago. At that time, there was a National Matching Plan, where, when one graduated from Medical School, one submitted an application for Internship, and one listed his or her first three choices in that order. I listed Cook County Hospital as my first choice. I was accepted there and trained in a Rotating Internship which was designed for one year. In addition, I stayed on, and took further training in certain specialities that I was interested in.

After entering practice in a rural area in Wisconsin, I was very grateful that I had had the experience of training at Cook County Hospital, a hospital of some 3300 beds in those days. The training was intense, comprehensive and involved training where we interns did so many procedures and interventions, under proper supervision, in so very many areas of medicine.

I often said, of the sixteen months at County, where I received room, board and $50 per month, that one never needed the room, because one was rarely in it. Somewhat of an exaggeration, but not much.

As stated above, I was to be so many times thankful for my training at County, where I had gained so much experience in so many areas, given the multitude of problems that I was to face later in my practice, where I was the one responsible for the care.

In a Rotating Internship, one spends times in many of the various specialities; Surgery, Internal Medicine, Pediatrics, Obstetrics, Gynecology, Orthopedics, Urology, etc. In all of these areas at County I received teaching in a great multitude of cases, including therapeutics and various intervention procedures, with appropriate supervision.

For example: on Obstetrical Service, I, myself, delivered over one hundred babies, including vaginal delivery of babies presenting in breech position. Vaginal delivery of "breech babies" was standard of care in those days. Also there were other complicated deliveries.

There was one Service at County called Pathologic OB, where women with some complications related to pregnancy were admitted. This included women in labor with other complications, such as having high fever, or other conditions which could complicate delivery. However, these were a minority of the reasons for admission to that Service. One of the main reasons was blood loss shock due to incomplete, spontaneous abortions (miscarriages). On that Service there was one physician on at a time, for twenty-four hours, then off for twenty-four hours. I served for one month on that Service.

Here is a more detailed example of my responsibilities on the Pathologic OB Service.

A young woman with an incomplete abortion (a spontaneous miscarriage), meaning there was still remnants of the pregnancy remaining in the uterus, that was causing the continued vaginal bleeding, would be admitted after presenting with significant blood loss, in a shock like condition. It was my job to quickly assess the situation, start an IV and do a quick blood count on the floor where we had a small lab, and where we, also, were the lab tech. If a blood transfusion was needed, which was almost always the case, we would personally take a blood specimen to the blood bank for type and cross match and when blood was ready, run to the blood bank to retrieve the blood and administer it to the patient. We would receive a number of these patients during each twenty-four shift. The problem was, they all had retained products of pregnancy in the uterus, which was causing the bleeding, and needed a "D & C" (dilation and curettage) a surgical procedure, where the uterus is emptied of this remaining tissue with surgical instruments. At the end of the twenty-four hour day, I did these in an area on the ward set up for that procedure. This was <u>after</u> my twenty-four shift, before leaving the ward. So by the end of the month, we, the other physician and myself, had each done a few dozen D & Cs.

In Surgery, we assisted on all types of cases, emergent and otherwise, and did several procedures ourselves, with appropriate supervision and assistance. I did tonsillectomies and an occasional appendectomy, etc. We were also highly involved with post-op care.

I took extra training in Anesthesia, where eventually I was giving anesthesia in several cases of general anesthesia, as well as spinal anesthesia.

In Pediatrics, I saw and cared for such a variety of serious problems, medical and surgical. I saw several cases of suspected meningitis, for example, where we often did the diagnostic spinal taps. Also shock, mainly as I recall, from dehydration due to acute gastroenteritis. Due to the hypotension accompanying these cases, I often had to do "cut downs" to gain venous access for fluid administration.

Internal Medicine was, as were all the services, extremely busy. I rotated on call, as well as serving during the day. We didn't get the day off after being on call. And admissions were such, that one was always up all night, the night on call. During the night on call I was responsible for new admissions, as well as any problems on my ward. And we had some sixty to eighty patients on each ward. A Resident in Internal Medicine was also available to assist, as needed. Again, I saw all types of medical problems, acute new problems such as myocardial infarctions, strokes, etc., as well as complications of chronic problems—chronic lung disease exacerbations, complications of diabetes, severe asthma attacks, etc. These were the days before Coronary Care Units and "ICUs."

In Ortho, I saw fractures of multiple kinds, and learned to reduce and cast these fractures. I assisted with Orthopedic surgery, such as hip fractures, fracture dislocation of the ankle, etc. I reduced dislocated shoulders, fingers, etc.

All the Services that I rotated on during our Internship at Cook County was very busy, as described above. There were so many procedures that I learned and did: Thoracentesis, Paracentesis, spinal taps (pediatric and adults), repair of all types of lacerations, starting all types of IVs in all types of patients, minor surgical procedures, as well as some major surgical procedures, as stated above.

I found, as stated above, my Internship at Cook County Hospital would serve me very well in my role as a primary physician, especially in a rural area, where significant help was often very limited or nonexistent.

A GENERAL DESCRIPTION OF THE MEDICAL COMMUNITY IN WISCONSIN DELLS IN 1960 AND FOR YEARS THEREAFTER

After October 1960, I joined three other physicians in practice at the Dells Clinic in Wisconsin Dells, Wisconsin. One of the physicians had surgical training.

Everyone did what General Practitioners did in those days, deliver babies, do some surgical procedures, depending on their training, cared for many types of fractures, minor trauma, infectious diseases of all kinds, took care of acute and chronic health problems, some emergent, including cardiovascular, pulmonary, gastrointestinal, endocrinology (including diabetes, thyroid and others), neurological, psychiatric issues, as well as the constant flow of acute and chronic, usually minor health problems—URIs, headaches, gastrointestinal problems, musculoskeletal problems, etc., etc., etc. I also assisted with surgery on my patients that were operated on by other surgeons and rendered the post-op care.

It was a robust, busy practice. There was no hospital in town, but patients were admitted to two hospitals in neighboring towns, one about ten miles and the other about fifteen miles away. I was on the Active Staff of both. Neither had an Emergency Room then, which was a factor, since Wisconsin Dells was a summer tourist destination and everything, including major and minor health problems, were brought to our clinic: heart attacks, diabetic complications, obstetric problems, auto accident victims, bee sting reactions, lacerations, fractures and all kinds of minor trauma, and many other major and minor problems. From Memorial Day through Labor Day, our clinic was open every day, including Saturdays, Sundays and Holidays. In addition, we made countless house calls to our own patients and to motels, campgrounds, etc., to see tourists. We rotated after-hours calls. One physician was on call at a time. During my first year in the Dells, I was on call for two nights of the weekdays, every other weekend and all the Holidays. The work load during the summer tourist season was nothing short of "brutal." But, after training at Cook County, I often said, "It seemed like a vacation." It really wasn't. There was no coronary care units, etc. Our ambulance was the old "hearse type," and the deputy police officer in town drove it when called. I did not have an unlisted phone number, and there was a local 24-hour establishment, who forwarded calls looking for a physician. Along with "tourist" demands, we also had a busy year-round practice. I had less of a general load initially, due to my just starting practice.

MORE SPECIFICALLY REGARDING MY INDIVIDUAL PRACTICE AT THE DELLS CLINIC, 1960s - ON

As time progressed, I began to build up a following of "my patients." I saw patients of all ages in outpatient practice at the clinic, for all kinds of problems that brought people to the doctor for care. I had privileges in both the hospitals in the neighboring towns, where our patients were admitted.

All physicians at the clinic followed their own patients in the hospital, making hospital rounds all days, including Saturdays, Sundays and Holidays, whether on call or not. We all delivered our own OB patients. Over the years I delivered hundreds of babies, including several with breech presentation. Vaginal delivery of "Breech Babies" was standard of care in the earlier days of my practice and I had had extensive training in that area. We all did some surgical procedures, depending on our training. Routine Tonsillectomies and Adenoidectomies, at about age five or six, was standard of care in those early days and I, personally, did a great number of these cases. I did an occasional D & C. But with one of my colleagues surgically trained, I did little else. I did assist in surgery on my patients requiring surgical procedures.

As mentioned above, I furnished Primary Care for a great variety of problems, including Myocardial Infarctions (heart attacks), strokes, infectious diseases of all types, reducing and casting fractures, repair of multiple types of lacerations, all types of injuries, acute diabetic problems (Diabetic Ketoacidosis, Hypoglycemia). Some things were more emergent than others. And in general, I saw and cared for the day-to-day types of things presenting to primary care in those days: complete physical exams, immunizations, screening tests, "minor" problems such as sore throats, earaches, URIs, viral infections, gastrointestinal problems, genitourinary problems, prenatal care, gynecological problems, dermatology issues, musculoskeletal complaints, pulmonary problems, psychiatric issues, and on and on.

A word further on one specific area—the repair of lacerations. I repaired hundreds of lacerations, minor, and some not so minor, year round, but so many during the summer tourist season. Also, fishing was a common recreational activity in the Dells area, in the Wisconsin River and in the many surrounding lakes. Over the years, I removed countless wayward, embedded fishhooks, from multiple body sites, especially during the tourist season.

A GAME CHANGER

First, a little background:

In the era referred to above, **heart attacks (myocardial infarctions)** were very common, and the mortality accompanying, was very significant. Often, the cause of death was **cardiac arrest**, so called "**sudden cardiac death.**" This was due to a fatal arrhythmia known as **ventricular fibrillation**, a situation where there is no effective heart muscle contraction to circulate blood. The result, unless reversed quickly, was death. This arrhythmia was not an uncommon occurrence in heart attacks, especially in the first few hours after onset of symptoms. Sometimes, cardiac arrest (sudden cardiac death) was the presenting symptom in a person who did not even realize they had heart disease. So, in those days, it was not uncommon to have a person collapse, unconscious, with no pulse or respiratory effort and be, in fact, dead. In my practice in the Dells, in the early years, I witnessed this a number of times. So mortality of heart attacks was significant in those days.

Discovery of the benefit of **CPR (cardiopulmonary resuscitation)** and **defibrillation** in the late 1950s and early 1960s as interventions in cases of cardiac arrest were SIGNAL events in the advance of medical science, and specifically in the treatment of heart attacks.

The following article will describe these events, which changed the care of the above described heart problems **(heart attacks, arrhythmias, sudden cardiac death, etc.)** across the nation and around the world.

The following is an article of the OSLER SOCIETY OF GREATER KANSAS CITY, recalling 50 years of acute coronary care.
(Published online at http://myoslersociety.sharepoint.com/Pages/CoronaryCareUnits.aspx, accessed January 18, 2015.)

50 Years of Acute Coronary Care

May 20, 2012 marked the 50th anniversary of the opening of the world's first coronary care unit, the Bethany Hartford Coronary Care Unit at Bethany Medical Center, Kansas City, Kansas. This simple but practical idea has saved thousands of lives and has added greatly to our knowledge of the electrical events that occur in an acute myocardial infarction. It also ushered in a new era for nurses where they became active participants in the treatment of patients.

If you were so unfortunate as to suffer a sudden cardiac arrest prior to 1956, your chances of survival were nil. The only thing that could be done for you was open chest cardiac massage. Not very convenient unless you were already under anesthesia on an operating room table.

Between 1956 and 1960, two major developments changed this dramatically. The first was the discovery by Jude, et al at John's Hopkins, that closed chest cardiac compression could effectively perfuse the body. The second was the discovery by Zoll, at Harvard, that the heart could be defibrillated with an external defibrillator. Neither of these developments alone would have been helpful, but together they provided an effective tool for the treatment of sudden cardiac arrest. This led to the development of the Crash Cart and the term Code Blue at Bethany Medical Center in 1960.

Within a few months every hospital had a Crash Cart. Early experience showed that unless CPR was begun within a minute or two of cardiac arrest the results were extremely poor. This led Dr Hughes Day and others at Bethany Medical Center to the idea of putting acute MI patients in close proximity to a monitor/defibrillator. Thus, was born the Coronary Care Unit.

Supported by a grant from the Hartford Foundation, the Bethany Hartford Coronary Care Unit was opened on May 20, 1962. The initial unit consisted of four private rooms and a seven bed open ward which was also used as a Medical Intensive Care Area. When a separate Medical Intensive Care Area was opened in 1970, the area was remodeled into a seven private bed unit.

Prior to 1962, the death rate from acute myocardial infarction among patients admitted to a general hospital was in the range of 30%. Today, every hospital has some kind of acute coronary care area and the mortality rate averages 3%.

Dr. Day has passed away and so has Bethany Medical Center, but his contribution will live forever. Rest well Hughes. You made a difference.

> Sherman M. Steinzeig, MD
> Medical Director,
> Bethany Hartford Coronary Care Unit
> 1969-1985

Following the above discoveries, several things changed locally in my practice area. Our community Hospital established a four bed "ICU," with monitoring and defibrillation capabilities. Heart attack patients were admitted there. In Wisconsin Dells, a volunteer "Rescue Squad" was formed. They were taught CPR (cardiopulmonary resuscitation) techniques (chest compression and respiration by face mask and bag).

I, myself, became certified in ACLS (Advanced Cardiac Life Support). To become certified, one had to demonstrate expertise in the use of the manual defibrillator (this was decades before the advent of the "automatic external defibrillator"), so common today. Also the proper use of various drugs used in the resuscitative protocol as well as insertion of an endotracheal tube to establish a more secure airway. I had already had extensive experience with this technique in my training at Cook County Hospital. We also had to know the basic CPR techniques. Written and Practical Exams had to be passed, and to maintain certification one had to pass the exams again, as there were changes in "protocols," every two years.

With the above changes in place, when someone collapsed, the volunteer rescue squad was called. They responded as quickly as possible and began CPR. Then, they frequently called me. I arrived at the scene, also as quickly as possible, finding CPR in progress. I quickly attempted defibrillation, which was almost always, and predictably, unsuccessful in restoring a pulse (indicating effective heart function).

Then I would start an IV, administer drugs, and repeat attempts at defibrillation, per protocol. Sometimes I would intubate the patient to establish better ventilation. These efforts were again almost always unsuccessful in resuscitating the patient. This was predictable, for to be successful, these interventions have to be applied in the first few minutes after arrest and there were unavoidable delays, given our situation.

The above scenario was repeated a number of times. However, when arrest occurred in an environment where these applications could be immediately applied, the outcome was significantly better. Later, when I describe in some detail some of the specific cases in which I was involved, this will be demonstrated.

THE FOLLOWING IS A PARTIAL LIST OF SOME OF THE MORE EMERGENT PROBLEMS THAT I ENCOUNTERED PERSONALLY, MULTIPLE TIMES, IN MY PRACTICE AT THE DELLS CLINIC, FOR WHICH I WAS RESPONSIBLE FOR THE DIAGNOSIS AND MANAGEMENT, COMPREHENSIVELY
OR AT LEAST, INITIALLY.
FOR THE MOST PART, I DID NOT ATTEMPT TO LIST THE MORE COMMON, LESS EMERGENT SITUATIONS ENCOUNTERED IN THE CATEGORIES BELOW.

Conditions highlighted in *bold italic* in the listings below are among the particular conditions or cases that I discuss in more detail in this work.

CARDIOVASCULAR PROBLEMS

Acute Myocardial Infarction (Heart Attack)
Cardiac Arrest ("sudden cardiac death")
Unstable Angina Pectoris
Stable Angina Pectoris
Hypertension
Congestive Heart Failure
(Systolic dysfunction)

(Diastolic dysfunction)
Acute Rheumatic Fever
Acute Pericarditis
Ruptured Thoracic Aortic Aneurysm
Ruptured Abdominal Aortic Aneurysm
Acute Pulmonary Embolism
Acute Arterial Embolism
(GI and Peripheral)
Ischemic Bowel Disease
Temporal Arteritis
Peripheral Artery Disease
Budd-Chiari Syndrome
Deep Venous Thrombosis
Ischemic and Chronic Venous Insufficiency
(Vascular Ulcers and Gangrene)

CARDIAC ARRHYTHMIAS

Ventricular Fibrillation
Torsade de Pointes
Ventricular Tachycardia
Accelerated Ventricular Rhythm
Ventricular Premature Contractions
Atrial Fibrillation
Atrial Flutter

Multifocal Atrial Tachycardia
Atrial Tachycardia
Paroxysmal Supra-Ventricular Tachycardia
Atrial Premature Contractions
Sinus Bradycardia
Asystole

HEART BLOCK

Sino-Atrial Block
First Degree A-V block
Second Degree A-V block
(Type 1 (Mobitz 1/Wenckebach))
(Type 2 (Mobitz 2))
Third Degree A-V block (complete heart block)

VALVULAR HEART DISEASE

Aortic Stenosis
Aortic Regurgitation
Mitral Stenosis
Mitral Regurgitation
Mitral Valve Prolapse

PRE-EXCITATION SYNDROMES

Wolff-Parkinson-White Syndrome

CONGENITAL HEART DISEASE

Atrial Septal Defect
Ventricular Septal Defect
Hypertrophic Cardiomyopathy
Patent Foramen Ovale
Long QT Syndromes

ACUTE STROKE

Ischemic
Hemorrhagic
Embolic
Cryptogenic
Subarachnoid Hemorrhage
TIAs

SHOCK

Hemorrhagic (blood loss)
Septic
Anaphylactic
(*stinging insects*, drugs)
Cardiogenic
Dehydration
Toxic Shock Syndrome

PULMONARY PROBLEMS

COPD (Chronic Obstructive Lung Disease)
(Chronic Bronchitis, Emphysema)
Asthma
Pulmonary Embolism
Spontaneous Pneumothorax
Traumatic Pneumothorax
Hemothorax
Hemoptysis
Pulmonary Hypertension
Acute Respiratory Distress Syndrome

GASTROINTESTINAL PROBLEMS

Zenker's Diverticulum
Gastro-esophageal Reflux
Bleeding Ulcerative Esophagitis
Bleeding Esophageal Varices
Dyspepsia
Peptic Ulcer
Bleeding Duodenal Ulcer
Perforated Gastric Ulcer
Ruptured Duodenum
Liver
(Cirrhosis, Hepatic Encephalopathy, Bleeding
Adenoma, Budd-Chiari syndrome)
Diverticular Bleeding
Common Duct Stones
Bowel Obstruction
(Adhesions, Hernia, Gallstone, Tumor)
Celiac Disease
Ulcerative Colitis
Rectal Prolapse
Thrombosed Hemorrhoids

GENITOURINARY PROBLEMS

Renal Insufficiency
(Acute, Chronic)
IGA Nephropathy
Alport Syndrome
Testicular Torsion
Stones
(Renal, Ureteral, Bladder)
Acute Urinary Retention
Obstructive Uropathy
(Stones, Prostate, Neurogenic)
Cancer
(Uterus, Cervix, Ovary)
Benign Ovarian Cysts
Ruptured Ovarian Cysts
Bleeding Ovarian Cysts
Uterine Bleeding
(Miscarriage, Dysunctional,Tumor)
Uterine Myomata (Fibroids)
Vaginitis
(Yeast, Bacterial Vaginosis,Trichomoniasis)

OBSTETRICAL PROBLEMS

Spontaneous Abortion (miscarriage)
Ectopic Pregnancy
Malposition
(*Breech*, occiput posterior)
Macrosomia
Shoulder Dystocia
Twins
Placenta Previa

NEUROLOGICAL PROBLEMS

Demyelinating Disorders
(*Multiple Sclerosis*)
Neurodegenerative Disorders
(Amyotrophic Lateral Sclerosis (ALS),
Parkinson's Disease)
Dementias
(Alzheimer's, Vascular, Lewy Body, Progressive
Supranuclear Palsy)
Parkinson's Disease
Impingement Disorders
(Cervical, Thoracic, Lumbar)
Seizures

(Grand Mal, Absence, Partial,
Partial Complex, Febrile)
Bell's Palsy
Neuropathies
(Ulnar Neuropathy, Carpal Tunnel Syndrome)
Neurolagias
(Post-Herpetic, Diabetic, Alcoholic,
B12 Deficiency, Ideopathic)
Traumatic Quadriplegia
Tremor
(Parkinson, Essential)
Epilepsy
(Ideopathic, Tumor, Trauma)

MUSCULOSKELETAL PROBLEMS

Osteoarthritis
Rheumatoid Arthritis
Reiter's Syndrome
Fractures
Central
(Skull, Facial, Vertebral (Cervical, Thoracic,
Lumbar), Pelvis, Rib)
Extremities

(Humerus, Radial Head, Radial Shaft, Colles,
Ulnar Shaft, Carpus, Carpal Navicular,
Metacarpals, Phalanges, Femur, Patella, Tibia,
Fibula, Tarsal, Metatarsals, Phalanges)
Dislocations
(Shoulder, Elbow, Patella, Ankle, Phalanges)
Cartilage, Ligament, Tendon Problems
(Rotator Cuff, Acromioclavicular,
Meniscus Knee (Medial, Lateral),
Medial Collateral, Wrist)
Sprains
(Ankle, Wrist)

ENDOCRINE PROBLEMS

Diabetes
(Type 1, Type 2)
Diabetic Ketoacidosis
Diabetic Hypoglycemic Coma
Hyperosmolar Non-Ketotic Coma
Thyroid
(Hyperthyroidism,
Hypothyroidism,
Thyroid Nodules, (Benign, Malignant))
Hyperparathyroidism

Adrenal
(Hyper (Cushing's Disease),
Hypo (Addison's Disease))
Ovary
(Polycystic Ovarian Syndrome,
Tumors (Benign, Malignant),
Cysts (Benign, Malignant, Ruptured))

OPHTHALMOLOGY PROBLEMS

Acute Narrow Angle Glaucoma
Open Angle Glaucoma
Conjunctivitis
(Viral & Bacterial)
Iritis
Foreign Bodies
Corneal Ulcers
Corneal Abrasions
Strabismus
Global Injuries
Hyphema
Hypopyon
Congenital Cataract

OTOLARYNGOLOGY PROBLEMS

Fractures
(Nasal, Facial, Mandibular)
Acute Nose Bleeds
(Anterior & Posterior)
Septal Perforations
Rhinitis
(Allergic, Vasomotor)
Nasal Polyps
Vestibular Dysfunction
(Benign Paroxysmal Positional Vertigo)
(Vestibular Neuronitis)
(Labyrinthitis)
(Meniere's Disease)
Tinnitus
(Multiple Causes)
Dysphagia
(Multiple Causes)
Obstructive Sleep Apnea

DERMATOLOGY ISSUES

Cancer
(Melanoma, Squamous cell, Basal cell)
Rashes
(countless kinds)
Acne Vulgaris
Rosacea
Psoriasis
Trauma
(lacerations, contusions)
Ingrown Toenails
Warts
Bites
Poison Ivy

PSYCHIATRIC DISORDERS

Major Depressive Disorders
Bipolar Disorder
(Type 1 and 2)
General Anxiety Disorder
Panic Attacks
Obsessive-Compulsive Disorder
Conversion Reaction

Psychotic Disorders
(Multiple Types)
(Acute and Chronic Schizophrenia)
Personality Disorders

INFECTIOUS DISEASE

CHILDHOOD DISEASES

Rubeola (red measles)
Rubella (german measles)
Mumps
Varicella (Chicken Pox)
Pertussis (Whooping Cough)
Erythema Infectiosum (Fifth Disease)
Roseola (Roseola Infantum)

CNS

Meningitis & Meningoencephalitis
(*Meningococcal Meningitis*)
(*Herpes Encephalitis*)
(Haemophilus Meningitis)
(*Mumps Meningoencephalitis*)
Tubercular Brain Abscess

CARDIOVASCULAR

Subacute Bacterial Endocarditis
Acute Pericarditis
Acute Rheumatic Fever

UPPER RESPIRATORY

URIs
Sinusitis
Pharyngitis
(Viral, Streptococcal, Yeast)
Peri-tonsillar Abscess
Oral Mucosa
(Yeast, Aphthous Ulcers, Herpes Simplex,
Coxsachie Virus (Hand, Foot and Mouth Disease)
Otitis Media
Malignant Otitis Media

PULMONARY

Tuberculosis
Pneumonia
(Viral, Aspiration, Bacterial
(Pneumococcal, Staphylococcal, Gram Negative,
Atypical, *Legionella*))

Lung Abscess
Empyema
Acute Exacerbations (COPD)
Bronchiectasis

GASTROINTESTINAL

Helicobacter Pylori
Viral Gastroenteritis
Salmonella Gastroenteritis
Giardiasis
Clostridia Difficile Diarrhea
Acute Cholecystitis
Acute Pancreatitis
Hepatitis
(*Hepatitis* A, B, *C*)
Subphrenic Abscess
Acute Appendicitis
Acute Diverticulitis
Rupturing Diverticulitis
Diverticular Abscess
Peri-rectal abscess

URINARY

Urinary tract infections
Uro-Sepsis
Pyelonephritis
Cystitis
Urethritis
(Gonococcal, Chlamydia, Trichomoniasis)

GYNECOLOGICAL

Mastitis
(Cellulitis, Abscess)
Pelvic Inflammatory Disease
(Gonococcal, Chlamydial, Multi-bacterial)
Cervicitis
Endometritis
Vaginitis
(Candidiasis, Bacterial Vaginosis, Trichomoniasis)

NEUROLOGICAL

Meningitis
(Meningococcal)
(Haemophilus)

Herpes Encephalitis
Herpes Zoster (Shingles)
Post Herpetic Neuralgia

MUSCULOSKELETAL, SOFT TISSUE

Toxic Shock Syndrome
Reiter's Syndrome
Cellulitis
(Staphylococcal, Methicillin Resistant
Staphylococcal, Strep, Multibacterial)
Necrotizing Fasciitis
(Flesh Eating Bacteria)
Osteomyelitis
Furuncles (boils)
Carbuncles
Infected Sebaceous Cysts

DERMATOLOGICAL

Erysipelas
Impetigo
Tinea Capitis
Tinea Corporis
Tinea Cruris
Tinea Pedis

Tinea Versicolor
Herpes Simplex
Herpes Zoster
Musculosum Contagiosum

INSECT VECTOR & PARASITIC

Ticks
(Lyme, *Babesosis*,
Ehrlichiosis/Anaplasmosis,
Rocky Mountain Spotted Fever)
Mosquito
(West Nile Virus)
Other
Scabies
Pediculosis Pubis
Pediculosis Capitis (Head Lice)
Swimmers Itch
Giardiasis
Pin Worms

SEXUALLY TRANSMITTED DISEASE

Gonorrhea
Chlamydia
Trichomoniasis

HIV
Pelvic Inflammatory Disease
Epididymitis
Herpes Simplex
Human Papilloma Virus
Genital Warts

CANCER

Brain
Lung
Thyroid
GI
(Oral, Esophagus, Gastric,
Colon, Colorectal, Carcinoid)
Pancreas
Liver
(Primary Hepatocellular, Metastatic)
Gall Bladder
Common Bile Duct
(Cholangio-Carcinoma)
GU
(Kidney, Bladder, Prostate)
(Uterus, Cervix, Ovary)
Breast

Bone
(Primary, Metastatic)
Skin
(Malignant Melanoma, Basal Cell, Squamous Cell)
Muscle
(Rhabdomyosarcoma)
Hematogenous
(Leukemias (many types), Multiple Myeloma)
Lymphomas
(Hodgkins, Non-Hodgkins)

ANEMIAS

Iron Deficiency
Acute Blood Loss
Hemolytic
Hemoglobinopathies
Pernicious (B12 Deficiency)
Chronic
(Kidney Disease, many others)
Cancer (many kinds)
Chemotherapy

AUTOIMMUNE DISORDERS

Ulcerative Colitis
Rheumatoid Arthritis
Disseminated Lupus Erythematosus
Sjogren's Syndrome
Sarcoidosis
Raynaud's Syndrome
Autoimmune Hepatitis
Autoimmune Thyroiditis
Giant Cell Arteritis

VASCULITIS

Many Types
(Infection, Drug, Genetic, Immune, Unknown)
Example: Temporal Arteritis

CONGENITAL DISORDERS

Congenital Heart Disease
Cystic Fibrosis
Hemochromatosis
Congenital Cataract
Anencephaly

Phenylketouria
Friedrich's Ataxia
Trisomy 21 (Down's Syndrome)
Mental Retardation (many causes)
Cerebral Palsy

ENVIRONMENTAL PROBLEMS

Hypothermia
Frostbite
Heat Stroke
Heat Exhaustion
Severe Sunburn
Poison Ivy
Swimmer's Itch

POISONINGS

Carbon Monoxide
Tylenol
Organic Nitrogenous Fertilizer
ManyTypes of Ingestions
(Chemicals, Drugs, Plants, Miscellaneous)

ADVERSE DRUG REACTIONS

Perforated Gastric Ulcer
Gastritis and Bleeding
Bleeding from Warfarin
(GI, Hematuria, Epistaxis, Thyroid, Hemarthrosis, Retroperitoneal)
Thrombocytopenia
Congestive Heart Failure
Hepatic Dysfunction
Nephrotic Syndrome
Angioedema
Oculogyric Crisis
Skin Rashes (multiple types)

The above list is far from complete, and some are not all that emergent, but gives one some flavor of the variety of problems that one encounters in primary care, either as "Gate Keeper," or, in most cases, for comprehensive management. At least that was my personal experience.

THE FOLLOWING ARE SOME SPECIFIC CASES THAT PRESENTED TO ME IN MY PRACTICE AT THE DELLS CLINIC THAT I WILL DESCRIBE IN SOME DETAIL

CASE NUMBER 1

This occurred rather soon after I began practice at the Dells Clinic in Wisconsin Dells in late 1960. I was "on call" this night, which was quite frequent during that first year, being the "junior" member of the four MDs of the clinic staff. This was in the evening after the clinic had closed. I received a call from parents of a rather young infant, perhaps, four to six months of age. They stated the infant had been crying, inconsolably, for some time, that evening. I received the call at my home (no unlisted number in those days). I arranged to meet the family at the clinic.

On arriving at the clinic, the infant was whimpering, crying and retracting the lower extremities. On questioning the parents, the infant had had no premonitory symptoms of any illness, including upper respiratory, pulmonary or gastrointestinal. The child was afebrile. The infant was not a patient of mine, but on questioning, there had been no history of abnormalities in the pregnancy, delivery, congenital problems or other concerns until now. Immunizations were up to date. Physical exam of eyes, ears, nose, throat, lungs and heart were within normal limits. However, on exam of the abdomen, I detected a small mass, palpable in the right mid-abdominal area.

Right away, I entertained a probable diagnosis of intussusception. Intussusception is a condition where the bowel, for a variety of reasons, can "telescope" into itself, causing an obstruction. This condition is a medical emergency and needs immediate intervention to relieve the obstruction. If allowed to persist, death in two to five days is a predictable outcome. I was familiar with this condition from my medical school training at the University of Illinois and my post graduate training at Cook County Hospital and realized the gravity of this problem and, indeed, if this diagnosis be correct, the need for emergent intervention, as it can lead to early fatal outcome if not corrected.

One of my partners was trained in General Surgery and did most of the surgical cases we had at the clinic. We had an X-ray machine at the clinic capable of fluoroscopy. I called my surgeon partner and he came to the clinic, examined the patient, and agreed with my suspected diagnosis. Next, we mixed up some Barium and proceeded to give the baby a Barium enema. We viewed it through the fluoroscope, and indeed, saw the intussusception at the terminal ileum and colon cecal area. It did not reduce with the pressure of the enema, which sometimes can happen.

We discussed the seriousness of the situation and the need for immediate surgical intervention with the parents. They agreed with the plan. The baby was transported to the hospital and the surgeon, with my assistance, performed a laparotomy, did the necessary procedure to correct the problem and prevent its recurrence.

I do remember the tiny appendix had been drawn into the intussusception and appeared inflamed and it was removed also.

The baby's post-op course was without incident.

CASE NUMBER 2

At another time, early in my career, I received a call to make a house call to see a boy of about sixteen who was ill with a fever.

On arriving, I discovered a youth who was quite somnolent with a high fever. He was somewhat responsive but definitely obtunded. His parents said he had complained of a headache. Exam revealed some stiffness of the neck (nuchal rigidity). He did not have many other significant physical findings except slight redness of his pharynx. Other than the fever, his vital signs (blood pressure, pulse, respiration) were normal. I was concerned with central nervous system infection (meningitis or meningoencephalitis) and asked the parents to take him to our local hospital.

On his arrival there, I immediately did a spinal tap. The spinal fluid appeared clear and normal. I ordered the usual evaluations of cell count, culture, protein, glucose, etc. Cell count revealed a number of white blood cells of the lymphocytic variety, consistent with a viral infection. Protein and glucose values were essentially normal.

I felt the patient had a viral meningo-encephalitis and started IV fluids, an antipyretic for fever and closely observed the patient's vital signs and sensorium. After several hours his sensorium seemed to be clearing and the next day his Parotid glands began to swell bilaterally. He had THE MUMPS, a known possible cause of meningo-encephalitis, but not commonly seen.

He had an uneventful recovery.

CASE NUMBER 3

In the early months, soon after I joined the Dells Clinic staff, I was on call and saw a young woman, complaining of pelvic pain. History revealed a missed menstrual period and some vaginal spotting. Exam revealed a palpable, tender mass in the right adnexal area and some lower abdominal tenderness. I suspected an ectopic pregnancy. This was in the days before ultrasound was available. The lady was a patient of the physician at the clinic who had surgical training, and who also did general practice, including obstetrical care. I called him and he came to the clinic, examined the patient, agreed with my diagnosis and determined she would need immediate surgery.

She was taken to our small community hospital in the next town and I also went there to assist with the surgery. On arrival, it was found that the nurse anesthetist was not available. I don't recall the actual reason. Another physician on the small active staff there volunteered that he could give "drop ether."

As mentioned earlier, I had had some training in anesthesia at Cook County Hospital in Chicago. In fact, I had given general, as well as spinal anesthesia, several times. I asked to see the nurse anesthetist's equipment.

Then, I said, I could administer a general anesthetic. This was agreed on, so we moved into the operating room and I proceeded to do just that, and my surgically trained partner did the surgery and, indeed, the patient did have an ectopic tubal pregnancy. Everything continued quite smoothly and the patient had an uneventful surgery and post-op recovery.

CASE NUMBER 4

During the early 1960s, acute myocardial infarctions were very common and mortality from such was very high, compared to today. Treatment modalities that made a difference were very limited. Complications of congestive heart failure, arrhythmias, including ventricular tachycardia and ventricular fibrillation were common and portended a bad prognosis, as to survival. Those were the days before the discovery and availability of CPR and defibrillation. Myocardial Infarctions (heart attacks) were admitted routinely to community hospitals, and care available at that time, administered, with often less-than-favorable outcome. The following describes one case under my care.

This was a gentleman who was retired but in generally good health and able to be normally active, until his heart attack. He was admitted, under my care, to our community hospital. EKG revealed an extensive anterior wall myocardial infarction. He quickly developed signs and symptoms of congestive heart failure and soon began to develop intermittent episodes of ventricular tachycardia, predicting very poor prognosis, as to survival. Pharmacologic interventions, in that time era, were very limited.

During that first night in the hospital, I sat at the patient's bedside, intermittently administering intravenously the drug, Procainamide, which had some known benefit in controlling ventricular tachycardia.

Unexpectedly, he improved and survived to leave the hospital.

However, he remained severely incapacitated with severe, chronic congestive heart failure (New York Heart Association Stage IV category, the worst category). I did continuing outpatient follow-up evaluations, including an EKG, that I saw was consistent with a left ventricular aneurysm.

In view of this, and his continuing disability, I contacted a cardiac surgeon in Madison whom I knew and discussed the case with him. Subsequently, the patient was referred and later underwent open heart surgery with resection of the aneurysm.

Over the next period of time, he improved dramatically, to where he was up and about and able to resume his normal activities. He was a retired carpenter by trade.

A footnote to this story: later I hired him to finish my basement.

CASE NUMBER 5

One summer day at the clinic, I was just finishing a busy morning and getting ready to leave for a quick lunch when, coming into the examining room area from the waiting room, I observed a young man being supported on either side by two other young men and being half-dragged and half-staggering to keep his feet. He appeared quite pale. The nurse that was accompanying them said to me, "He's been stung by a bee."

He was placed on an exam table in the nearest room by his friends. He was very weak and barely able to talk. His skin was cool and clammy and he was very pale. His pulse was rapid and weak. He had a few scattered urticarial lesions (hives). His blood pressure was barely obtainable. He complained of feeling short of breath but, on examining the lungs, no definite rales could be appreciated. He was experiencing an anaphylactic allergic reaction to venom from a stinging insect.

I had called immediately for my nurse to get the epinephrine and oxygen and I immediately administered a dose of epinephrine. I had also called for an IV setup and an ambulance, given his serious condition. While the ambulance was en route to the clinic, I had started and IV, given an IV dose of Solu-Medrol (a corticosteroid), and prepared a dilute solution of epinephrine to give intravenously.

I then accompanied him in the ambulance, administering the IV epinephrine and monitoring his condition during the trip to our local hospital, and I stayed with him in the ICU until his signs and symptoms began to improve and stabilize. He spent the remainder of the day and overnight in the ICU and was discharged the next day with an Epi-Pen with instructions and advice to see an allergist in about six weeks for a detailed workup with a goal of desensitization.

Over the years, I saw many more cases of generalized reactions to stinging insects, but the above was one of the more severe that I recall.

CASE NUMBER 6

For several years, the active staff at St. Clare Hospital rotated call to care for patients admitted through the emergency room, who did not have a local physician. Some of the more memorable cases that were admitted to my service come to mind.

One afternoon, while seeing my schedule of outpatients at the Dells Clinic, I received a call stating a tourist patient with a persisting headache was being admitted. She had been to the ER about three times over several hours with an unrelenting headache and treatments prescribed had not been successful in giving relief. Her home was in another state. The ER physician said he had even called the patient's physician at her home, and he had not been unduly concerned, as apparently she suffered from frequent headaches. He had some suggestions, but nothing that had been done, had resulted in any significant relief. The ER physician indicated the patient seemed to be stable otherwise, with normal vital signs, and in no significant serious distress of any kind, but felt she needed to be admitted for further care.

I received no additional calls from the hospital regarding the patient's condition. It was near the end of the day when I had received the call from the ER, and two or three hours later, I arrived at the hospital to check the patient and assume care. The nursing staff had not called with any concerns regarding the patient in the interim.

On walking into the room, looking at the patient lying in bed, several very concerning signs presented to me. The patient was very somnolent, and as I observed her, she was having Jacksonian (march) seizures, beginning with muscular twitching of one side of the face, then progressing to jerking and twitching of an upper extremity. This was consistent with a significant intracranial problem.

The patient was quite obtunded, and it was difficult to get any meaningful history. I did a quick neurological exam which was not really very revealing as to etiology, although several possible diagnoses existed. The patient's respiratory effort also was declining to an extent that was very concerning.

I felt with this presentation, it was imperative that she be in a center where more specialized intervention, diagnostic and therapeutic, would be available. I quickly called a neurologist on call at a hospital in Madison, that we often referred to, spoke briefly with him, and he said, "Why don't you bring her down?"

In that early year, there was no real transport mechanism to transfer patients in unstable condition such as respiratory distress. Also, our hospital did not have a respirator at that time. So, next, I called one of our nurse anesthetists, explained to him the problem, and asked him to come in. I told him she needed to be transferred but this could not be done safely without respiratory support. I had called the local ambulance, which was standing by.

On his arrival, I told the anesthetist we would need to intubate the patient and accompany her in the ambulance and "bag" her (assist her respiration effort) on the way down. So we quickly intubated the patient and rode with her in the ambulance, supporting her respiration. The trip took about forty-five minutes to an hour. We arrived without further incident, with the remainder of the patient's vital signs remaining stable as they had been on our departure. She was admitted there and care was transferred to the receiving hospital.

    I did not receive frequent updates of her condition there, but later learned she remained hospitalized and expired some two to three weeks later. Her final diagnosis was HERPES ENCEPHALITIS.

CASE NUMBER 7

The dismal lack of success of resuscitative efforts performed in the community in cases of cardiac arrest, described previously, are in contrast to the often successful effort when defibrillation was done without delay, as depicted in the following two incidents.

One summer day, on a weekend, I was on duty at the clinic, along with my nurse. During summertime in the Dells, the town had many tourists and the downtown area was filled with people visiting the various shops, taking scenic boat rides on the river, etc.

The ambulance brought a patient to the clinic from the downtown area, where they had been called. He was complaining of chest pain. He had symptoms consistent with coronary ischemia. After a brief exam, I instructed the ambulance crew to take him to the hospital located about ten miles away in the next town, where we had recently created a small "ICU." When they were just loading him onto the gurney for placement into the ambulance, he "coded" (CARDIAC ARREST).

At that time, there was a manual defibrillator in the ambulance (this was years, of course, before the automatic external defibrillators became available). We, at that time, did not have a defibrillator at the clinic. I asked the ambulance driver to quickly get it, which he did. I immediately charged it and administered one shock and the patient immediately responded, going back into sinus (normal heart) rhythm and quickly regained consciousness. I accompanied him to the hospital and got him set up there.

I learned he was a patient of an MD whose practice was in the town where the hospital was located, so his ongoing care was turned over. I learned that some time later he had been transferred to the University Hospital in Madison, where he underwent bypass surgery.

CASE NUMBER 8

In the early morning hours, while I was still at home, I received a call (no unlisted number in those days) from the spouse of a family that lived in the country that I cared for. She reported her husband had suddenly become ill and she described symptoms consistent with an acute myocardial infarction (heart attack).

I instructed her to take him immediately to the hospital where I would meet them. I met them on arrival at the hospital and admitted him to one or our "ICU"-monitored beds. We had just recently established a four-bed "ICU" with monitoring and defibrillation capability. An immediate EKG revealed changes of an acute inferior wall myocardial infarction (heart attack). By this time, his symptom of chest pain had largely abated.

I began completing a history and physical exam. Then, as I began a brief abdominal exam, I heard a gurgle, looked up to find him unresponsive and the monitor showing ventricular fibrillation ("sudden cardiac death"). I quickly asked the patient's wife, who was at his bedside, to step out into the hallway and called for the nurse to bring the defibrillator. Quickly, after charging, I placed the paddles, administered one shock, and immediate sinus (normal heart) rhythm was restored. The patient quickly regained consciousness and was responding as if nothing had occurred. I'm not sure if he ever was quite aware of what had happened. Most assuredly, fortunate timing for him.

When I left the Dells, some thirty years later, he was still up and about and functioning normally.

During my time in the Dells, and at the community hospital where we admitted and cared for our patients, they were several "codes" (cardiac arrests). Intervention was sometimes successful, sometimes not.

CASE NUMBER 9

One evening, I received a call at home from our local nursing home, where I had several patients as residents. This patient of mine had been there for some time. She had Multiple Sclerosis and was essentially paralyzed from the waist down, and had a permanent indwelling foley catheter in her urinary bladder.

I was told she was ill, so I went to the home to check on her. I found her in serious condition. She was somewhat somnolent, febrile, with a rapid pulse and very low blood pressure. Rapid exam revealed no definite site of infection and I suspected she was in a septic shock condition from urosepsis (urinary tract infection that had spread into the blood stream). Septic shock carried a high mortality in those days, and in fact, still does. I called the ambulance and had her transported to the hospital where I arrived at the same time to provide further care.

I quickly established an IV and began rapid IV fluid administration, along with broad spectrum IV antibiotic coverage. I obtained blood and urine specimens for culture, and other appropriate studies.

About that time, the patient had a grand mal seizure. She had no prior history of seizures. She had no definite physical signs of central nervous system infection. I immediately obtained a "spinal tray," turned the patient on her side in her bed and did a lumbar puncture. The spinal fluid appeared "normal", and the initial tests on the spinal fluid were within normal limits. The culture result, when eventually returned, showed "no growth."

The patient received several liters of IV fluid during her first few hours in the hospital, as well as transient use of a vasopressor drug to support her blood pressure. Blood and urine cultures were later reported positive for bacterial infection. She gradually showed signs of improvement and eventually recovered to her pre-hospital state and returned to the nursing home.

A case of SEPTIC SHOCK, which carries a significant mortality.

CASE NUMBER 10

Another case, I recall, was an adult gentleman, about sixty years of age, who came into my examining room with nonspecific symptoms, stating he had just been "not feeling well" for some time. He stated also that he had been having a fever, on and off. He generally felt weak and unwell. On exam, it was noted he had a low grade fever, appeared a bit pale and did appear to be ill. Pulse rate was more rapid than would be accounted for by his slight temperature elevation. Further findings included a systolic heart murmur, louder at the cardiac apex and radiating to the left axillary area, consistent with mitral regurgitation (valvular heart disease). Lungs were clear. In addition, on oral exam, a severe pyorrhea was noted.

I began to suspect a subacute bacterial endocarditis. However, I did not note any Roth spots, Osler nodes or Janeway lesions, often seen with that condition. I don't recall now what his urinalysis revealed. I drew blood cultures and these were eventually returned as positive for strep viridans, a bacteria that is commonly found among the bacterial organisms found in the mouth. If it gets into the blood stream, it can be the cause of endocarditis. Cultures for strep viridans are often positive in blood cultures in subacute bacterial endocarditis.

Due to the nature of the case and lengthy treatment required, if indeed this was the diagnosis, I wished confirmation. So I referred the patient, along with the above information, to a cardiologist that I knew, and he agreed with the diagnosis and outlined what he thought was appropriate treatment, which included long term intravenous antibiotics. This led to the patient's admission to our local nursing home where this treatment was carried out without incident. Eventually he made a complete recovery.

CASE NUMBER 11

One morning, while still at home, I received a call from the mother of a family that I cared for, stating her daughter, about sixteen years of age, was quite ill. She was rather nonspecific as to detail, but said she had been complaining of an upset stomach and abdominal pain, and had become very weak and seemed very sleepy. The mother also said she and her husband had to be in court quite early for a proceeding which they could not delay. I instructed them to take her to our local hospital and I called the hospital to have her admitted, telling them I would be there without delay.

On entering the room where the daughter had been admitted shortly before, I was immediately aware of a serious problem. She was resting in bed, on her back, quite somnolent, and with obvious Kussmaul respiration. That is, with deep, slow and long inspiration and expiration. This type of respiration is seen in conditions where the blood is acidotic. I suspected diabetic ketoacidosis. The child was not a known diabetic.

I immediately ordered tests, including blood sugar, electrolytes, etc., moved her into our "ICU," started an IV and began rapid fluid administration. Test results, returned shortly thereafter, revealed a blood sugar of around one thousand, as I recall (normal fasting blood sugar is under one hundred). IV insulin was begun. I drew an arterial blood gas, that showed a pH of 6.9 (normal 7.35-7.45), the lowest I had ever seen. She had a case of very severe diabetic ketoacidosis—a very serious condition, associated with significant mortality.

I remained at the hospital all that day, administering IV insulin and fluids and monitoring her vital signs and electrolytes and blood sugar. I stayed at the hospital that entire night also, continuing to monitor the above and managing her treatment. She required, along with a large volume of IV fluid, very large amounts of IV potassium. She also developed other very worrisome problems of intermittent ventricular tachycardia.

In these early years of my practice in Wisconsin Dells, the lab at our small community hospital was normally closed at night. I requested one of the lab techs to stay through the night, which they did. In those days, lab evaluations were considerably more labor intensive and I was ordering blood sugars, electrolytes, etc., almost hourly. By the time one set of results were completed, another sample was being submitted. Her condition and lab results gradually improved during the night, and by morning of the next day, twenty-four hours after admission, she was much improved.

In due time, her diabetes came under adequate control. Later, she married, and became the mother of a couple of healthy infants.

CASE NUMBER 12

As mentioned before, the active staff at our small community hospital rotated call to accept and care for patients who were admitted to the hospital through the emergency room and had no local physician.

Late one day, when I was finishing by schedule at the clinic, I received a call that a patient was being admitted to my service. The patient was a teenage boy from the Chicago area, who was with a group having an outing at a local park. They had been playing Frisbee. In that park there were steel grills for public use, imbedded in a concrete base. The youth had been running, looking back and had impacted one of these grills with his abdomen.

Subsequently, he developed unrelenting abdominal pain and was taken to the hospital emergency room, where he was examined. Tests were done without coming up with a diagnosis. Vital signs were stable and abdominal exam was unrevealing and blood studies and x-rays were unremarkable. This was before ultrasound and CT scans were in use.

Soon, I finished at the clinic, and traveled to the hospital. I found the patient in about the same state with normal vital signs, and an abdominal exam that was non diagnostic. Blood tests of CBC, pancreatic enzymes, liver function tests, etc., were all within normal limits. However, the patient was continuing to complain of abdominal pain. This was about nine, or so, in the evening and I instructed the nurse on duty to call me in two hours with an update, and I returned home.

The nurse did as instructed. She stated, in a rather matter of fact manner, the patient was still complaining of abdominal pain and otherwise his condition was unchanged. His vital signs, blood pressure and pulse, remained unchanged. However, praise be to God, before hanging up, she added, "But now, he also is complaining of pain in his right testicle."

I immediately felt I knew what was wrong. I jumped out of bed, went to the hospital and indeed his exam had changed. Now on palpation in the right upper quadrant of his abdomen and flank, a crackling sensation was felt, consistent with subcutaneous emphysema (air in the tissue below the skin). His diagnosis, I felt, was a ruptured duodenum, a very serious problem that requires emergent surgical intervention. Anatomically, the duodenum lies retroperitoneal, and the air and fluid leak had caused irritation about the right kidney and ureter and he was experiencing referred pain to the right testicle.

I did not feel the surgical intervention he required was available locally. Quickly, I had an ambulance summoned, called the University Hospital in Madison, discussed the situation with the appropriate providers there, and sent him down. He underwent surgery soon after arrival that night, and indeed, he did have a ruptured duodenum.

As a footnote, after the above arrangements were made, I was able to talk to his mother in Chicago. I learned she, herself, was an ICU nurse there.

CASE NUMBER 13

One weekend day, I was home and received a call from a mother of a family that I cared for, calling regarding one of her children, a teenage daughter. She stated she was quite ill with a high fever and wondered if I might "call something in" to the drugstore for her. On further questioning, she told me the child had been complaining of a headache, and then she volunteered, "I think she might be coming down with the measles," because she had noted a rash. I knew the child had had the red measles vaccine. So I told the mother I would meet them at the clinic.

After seeing the child, I immediately became quite concerned. She indeed had a fever and complained of a headache. She seemed rather somnolent also but able to respond slowly to my requests. On her chest and abdomen, a few scattered skin lesions of small, erythematous, somewhat vesicular papules were visible. On exam I detected a bit of nuchal rigidity (stiff neck). I immediately thought she had meningococcal meningitis and realized the seriousness, especially in this case, with the skin lesions, which were probably a sign of Waterhouse-Friderichsen syndrome being present, a severe form of the above with an associated bacteremia, and associated with a significant mortality.

I felt with the time necessary to get the patient hospitalized locally, get antibiotics started, etc., I could have the patient in Madison almost as quick. So I called a Pediatrician I knew, discussed the case, and had her on her way. Indeed, other tests done there confirmed the diagnosis of meningococcal meningitis.

Fortunately, she did very well, and recovered without any residual neurological deficits. I was so glad the mother had mentioned "the measles."

One never knew what is going to show up next, for which one is responsible.

CASE NUMBER 14

Another patient that I became involved with was an eighty-plus year-old lady, who lived in a small neighboring town. She came to the clinic with a history and symptoms of rectal pathology and exam and tests led to a diagnosis of colorectal cancer. My surgical partner was consulted and she was admitted to the hospital, underwent further evaluation and then underwent surgery. Primary anastomosis was accomplished and the patient did not require a colostomy. Due to her advanced age and generally frail condition, she was discharged to the nursing home located in our clinic area and I was to manage her post-op care.

Quite soon, she developed a cough. With other concerning symptoms being present, I did a workup and sputum exams were done and were positive for acid fast bacteria, consistent with pulmonary tuberculosis. Cultures would later confirm pulmonary tuberculosis. Immediate action was required, especially given the nursing home environment. This happening in a nursing home environment created many problems of further testing of a multitude of other nursing home residents, besides arranging treatment for the patient. I discussed referral with the patient for specific treatment of her disease but she adamantly refused to be transferred anywhere and insisted that I take care of her.

Consequently, she was discharged to her home, which, as previously mentioned, was a short distance away in a neighboring small town, where she lived with her elderly husband. I involved the County Nurse, who discussed other treatment options with the patient, but she still refused any movement to any treatment facility.

So I did assume the treatment myself, starting her on a four-drug regimen. I thoroughly discussed with her the possible side effects and how we would monitor her. So I made many house calls. I used a mask, gowned and gloved, on the many visits to her home. I examined the patient, drew any necessary blood tests while there, and transported the samples to the lab. The patient did develop side effects to some of the medications, requiring changes in her regimen, but gradually improved and eventually made a complete recovery, with negative cultures of sputum specimens.

She was still coming to the clinic for checkups for other health problems when I finally left years later.

CASE NUMBER 15

One evening, when just the nurse and I were on duty at the clinic, a patient came in complaining of a backache which was of very recent onset. He seemed to be in some distress. He was just passing through our area and was staying at a motel in the area. He had few other symptoms and no good history pointing to the etiology of his complaints. He was a retired airline pilot, in his sixties, as I recall, and had no significant health problems.

Exam was rather unremarkable, with normal vital signs, normal blood pressure, normal pulses, including femoral and lower extremity pulses. Exam of heart, lungs and back also was within normal limits. His abdominal exam was unremarkable as to masses, or organomegaly. He had no flank tenderness. Urinalysis was negative for microscopic hematuria, which might suggest "kidney stones." As mentioned, he seemed in enough distress that I advised admission to the hospital for further exam, tests and monitoring. He said, "I'm not going to any hospital. Just give me something for pain. If I get worse, I will call you." So, he left the clinic.

A few minutes later, I heard a siren in Lake Delton, another small community with common border to Wisconsin Dells. They had a rescue squad of "First Responders." Right away I got a call, asking if I had just seen this patient, and I answered affirmatively. They said that his wife was driving him back to their motel in Lake Delton and he had become nauseated, got out of the car, and collapsed. I instructed them to take him immediately to the hospital. I called the hospital, told them to admit him and I would be there at once.

I drove there at once, and they had just moved him into a room. I immediately was aware of the problem. The patient was pale, skin clammy, and I noted some abdominal distension. He had a rapid, hardly palpable pulse, and his blood pressure was difficult to obtain. I was aware he had a ruptured abdominal aortic aneurysm. Often the outcome is sudden death.

I requested the nurses to quickly get me equipment to start an IV, but the patient had no signs of venous access anywhere, given his severe hypotensive condition. I requested "cut down" instruments and with a scalpel opened up the ante-cubital areas at the elbows bilaterally to gain access to the larger veins located there. Then I quickly secured venous access in both areas. I drew blood, sent it to the lab for typing and requested blood of his type immediately, without taking time for a cross-match.

I had also requested an ambulance be called during these proceedings. The ambulance responded quickly. We loaded the patient without delay. I took along a supply of blood of his type which had, however, not been cross-matched. The blood was in plastic containers and I had hung a unit on each IV. I wrapped a blood pressure cuff around each unit, pumped up the pressure to force the blood in faster. I had called the University Hospital in Madison of the situation. We arrived there with the patient's blood pressure somewhat better but the patient was still very hypotensive.

On arrival, a resident in Vascular Surgery was there to meet us. He quickly examined the patient and began making the arrangements for emergency surgery. While doing this, he had sent the patient to an adjoining area for a quick cross-table lateral x-ray of the abdomen to check for a calcium configuration that sometimes could be seen in abdominal aortic aneurysms (this was in the days before Ultrasound and CT). I remember the resident's name was Dr. Sam ----.

They were just loading the patient on a gurney to take him to the operating room, when a tech from X-ray came into the room and said, "Dr. ----, the Radiologist says he can see no signs of an aneurysm." Then I recall Dr. Sam saying, "To hell with that, get him up to the OR."

I learned later that he survived.

Footnote: The next summer, when I was away for a few days vacation, the Dells Clinic staff said this patient stopped by the clinic to see me. But we never saw each other again. I jokingly said, "He probably wanted to complain about the scars on his arms."

CASE NUMBER 16

Another case I will describe is an elderly man with multiple chronic health problems, chronic lung disease and diabetes, whom I entered into the hospital with a high fever and physical and radiographic signs of pneumonia. He was quite ill, and I started him on antibiotics recommended by CDC guidelines for the treatment of community acquired pneumonia (intravenous Ceftriaxone and Azithromycin). He was on oxygen and other interventions, as he required.

Despite this treatment, over the next couple of days his condition worsened and continued to deteriorate. The outcome was definitely in doubt. The medications mentioned were designed to cover multiple causes of pneumonia, including the more common pneumococcal and other gram-positive and gram-negative bacterial causes, and some of the more common atypical causes, including mycoplasma, chlamydia, legionella, etc.

I had obtained blood and sputum cultures of admission, as well as a urine specimen for Legionella antigen. This later test was only moderately sensitive for picking up Legionella pneumonia, but if positive was quite specific (confirmatory). This test result had not been returned. With the patient's condition deteriorating, I decided to empirically change his antibiotic regimen. So I switched him to a different antibiotic, Levofloxacin, which had just recently become available. It had a broad spectrum of activity against a wide range of bacteria, including atypicals, and specifically, had very good activity against Legionella bacteria.

Within twenty-four hours the patient's temperature defervesced and he began to improve. A bit later, the test result on the urine specimen for legionella antigen returned and it was positive. He had Legionella pneumonia, so-called Legionnaire's Disease.

He went on to recover to his pre hospital state.

CASE NUMBER 17

Another example of one never knows what will show with the next patient:

One summer afternoon at the Dells Clinic, a family brought in their young child who had been ill for a short time with a fever. The child had also complained of a headache and had not been feeling well at all, and did appear ill. They had been vacationing in the West in the Rocky Mountains and were on their way home to the eastern United States.

As I recall, exam did not point to a specific etiology. However, I had noted an erythematous, maculopapular rash on the child's distal forearms and hands. With this finding, I considered Rocky Mountain Spotted Fever being definitely in the differential diagnosis, even though they gave no definite history of recent tick bites. This type of rash is rather typical of that disease. With this disease, it is very important to begin treatment early, as there is significant mortality if treatment is delayed. Also, tests to confirm the diagnosis take time and, if the diagnosis is suspected, treatment with the indicated antibiotic should be begun.

I discussed my concerns with the family and after discussion, I called physicians at the University Hospital in Madison, who agreed to see the child promptly on arrival there, and the family departed for there, about a forty-five minute trip. I really don't know all the procedures and treatment she received there, but I know they were definitely concerned with that diagnosis also. Additional tests and treatment were carried out there.

CASE NUMBER 18

During my early years at the Dells Clinic, it was rather routine that young children, five or six years of age, underwent Tonsillectomy and Adenoidectomy. I had been trained in this procedure, and during that time probably did seventy-five to a hundred cases. I never had a significant complication or never had to return a patient to the operating room for post op bleeding, etc. I would see the child for a pre-op history and physical and admit them to the hospital one evening, do the surgery the next morning and they would stay in the hospital that day, and be discharged the first post-op day, if everything was going well.

It was common practice in those days to use intramuscular Codeine for pain in these post-op cases. One day, I had done one of these cases, and returned to the clinic and was seeing my regular schedule of patients. The nurse on duty at the hospital, who was doing the post-op care, called me and said she had made a mistake, and had given my patient Morphine rather than Codeine. Morphine, of course, is a much more potent drug.

Realizing the seriousness of this, I immediately returned to the hospital and did find the young child developing significant respiratory depression. I started an IV and administered intravenous Narcan (a drug that rapidly reverses the action of Morphine). There was very rapid improvement in the respiratory effort of the patient. However, knowing the short half-life (duration of effect) of Narcan (compared to the longer half-life of Morphine), I remained at the patient's bedside and administered additional doses of Narcan as required when symptoms of respiratory depression recurred. I did this until the patient's respiration remained normal.

I was so pleased that the nurse noted her error and was not hesitant to make it known to me.

CASE NUMBER 19

One night in my early time at the Dells Clinic, I was on call and got a call that there had been a motor accident in the area, and I was summoned to the scene. This was common practice in my early days—that I would get a call to go to an accident scene and be the only medical personnel there. This happened on a number of occasions, sometimes when there were multiple injuries, some being serious.

On this occasion, I arrived at the scene and found a young man bleeding from multiple, deep, transverse lacerations across the lower face, neck and upper chest. The story was that he was asleep in the backseat of a car which struck the rear of another vehicle that was parked alongside the highway. He was ejected through the windshield. An ambulance had been called.

Having my bag and some supplies, I used gauze pads and a couple of elastic bandages and wrapped the area of the neck and face. We arrived at our local community hospital (no emergency room in those days). A more thorough exam of the youth revealed no other serious injuries. Then, with the help of one of the Sister nurses (nuns) there, I proceeded to cleanse the wounds and painstakingly repaired the lacerations, one after the other, which was a lengthy process. The patient was kept in the hospital until his condition was appropriate for discharge to return to his home in an adjoining state for follow-up care.

A few months later, I received a nice letter from his mother, thanking me, and telling me how nicely his lacerations had healed.

CASE NUMBER 20

I had an elderly lady in my practice whom I had seen on an occasional basis. She also had advanced osteoarthritis, for which she was seeing an Internal Medicine Specialist, in another city. At his direction, she had been for some time, on regular doses of an NSAID drug (non steroidal anti-inflammatory drug); example: (ibuprofen). One known side effect of this class of drugs, of course, was upper gastrointestinal problems (ulcers, bleeding, etc.).

I received a call one night from her son, who stated his mother was complaining of rather severe abdominal pain and requested I come to her home, which I did. She stated the pain had started suddenly and she had not been having any "stomach trouble" at all, before this night. Examination revealed definite signs of significant peritonitis (a very tender-to-the-touch and firm abdomen). I had her taken to our community hospital and immediately got a series of blood tests and plain x-rays of the abdomen. The x-rays revealed free air in the abdominal cavity.

I summoned our surgeon, who examined the patient, and that night we took her to the operating room. Laparotomy revealed a *huge* (the largest I had ever seen) perforated gastric ulcer. She had a somewhat stormy course in the hospital post operatively, but was finally discharged to a local nursing home.

Addendum:

In my early years of practice, I had seen patients with other serious side effects of NSAIDs, (upper GI bleeding requiring transfusions, renal injury causing nephrotic syndrome). I never saw a fatality due to NSAIDs, but I seldom prescribed this class of drugs to elderly patients, who are more susceptible to the adverse effects of this class of medication. When I did prescribe this class of medicines, I did so for only a very brief time. Also, it was well known that serious upper GI adverse problems can develop without warning symptoms.

CASE NUMBER 21

One morning at the clinic I was seeing a local high school student for a complaint, the details of which I don't recall. At the end of her appointment, she shared with me a concern she had for a friend, a female classmate. She stated her friend had been upset about some issue the evening before, and had taken a large overdose of Tylenol, perhaps a whole bottle.

Aware of the seriousness of this, I made some calls to the girl's parents and got her into the clinic. She was not very symptomatic at the time, but being aware of the seriousness of this overdose and the usual delay in onset of symptoms in Tylenol poisoning, I immediately hospitalized her. A blood specimen was obtained for various tests, including blood levels of acetaminophen (Tylenol). We knew the approximate time of ingestion, so we could utilize the acetaminophen nomogram to assess more accurately the prognosis and need for emergent treatment, which included the drug, N-acetylcysteine. Also, liver function tests were drawn. The AST and ALT (liver transaminases) normally have an upper limit of normal around forty or fifty. When liver cells are injured by infection, alcohol, etc., these values rise. Usually, in an alcoholic or in someone with acute hepatitis, they rise significantly, but not to the extent found in this case. My patient's results were in the thousands.

Results of the acetaminophen nomogram indicated the need for treatment. N-acetylcysteine was indicated, which is given orally. I tried to start acetylcysteine, an antidote for Tylenol, orally, but the patient seemed reluctant and somewhat intolerant. After a bit of discussion, I was able to insert a nasogastric tube and began administering the drug by that route.

In the meantime, I had personnel contacting the University Hospital for me, as I wished to transfer the patient there as soon as possible. At that point, I wasn't sure that the youth would not need an emergent liver transplant, which sometimes is needed in serious Tylenol poisoning. After I discussed the situation with them, they, of course, were quite willing to accept the patient, and transfer was accomplished. Treatment was continued there, including the above drug, and eventually the patient made a complete recovery with no significant residual.

CASE NUMBER 22

One evening during my early months in the Dells, when I was on call, I received a call at home from a lady saying her elderly mother, who was a bit frail but still lived alone, was ill, and she requested a house call. It was during the winter months.

The patient's daughter was there when I arrived. The patient had become ill that evening, complaining of a headache, feeling a bit dizzy and weak. There were influenza cases in the community. After checking the patient, I found no outstanding signs of concern and felt she was probably "coming down with a virus of some type." I shared this with the daughter and returned to my home which was only about three blocks away.

Not long after returning home, the daughter called again, saying she thought she was getting the "same thing," because now she was getting a headache, and feeling a bit dizzy also. THE LIGHTS WENT ON! CARBON MONOXIDE POISONING!

I immediately hurried back to the house and opened the door and had the daughter open the windows. It was cold outside. It was an old dwelling, and the furnace was in a small basement. I had called a worker from the gas company that I knew and expressed my concern, and he came quickly. He had some sort of colorimetric test to detect carbon monoxide. He descended into the area where the furnace was located and almost immediately shouted, "Help me out of here!" I reached down, but he really didn't need any help, as he exited the area quite expediently on his own.

As the daughter's house was just down the street, a block away, we bundled up the mother, sat her on a stool chair, and the gas company worker and I carried her down the street to the daughter's house.

CASE NUMBER 23

One evening, when I was on call at home, I received a call from the local "Rescue Squad" who said they were bringing in an unresponsive individual. I met them at the clinic on their arrival.

The gentleman was not a patient of mine, but I recognized him as a cook at one of the local dinner houses I frequented. While I was not intimately acquainted with his health problems, I did know he was a diabetic. He, indeed, was in an unresponsive state, not responding to any verbal stimuli.

I presumed he was most likely in a severe hypoglycemic state, given his diabetic condition. His vital signs were unremarkable otherwise, and a brief physical exam gave no clue as to other possible causes. So I immediately got a vial of concentrated glucose solution for IV use, which we kept on hand for exactly this problem, and administered it IV.

He very quickly began to respond and soon became aware of his surroundings. He recognized me and then he said, "Hey Doc, I haven't seen you for a while. When are you going to come out for a fish fry?" That got a few chuckles and comments from the guys on the Rescue Squad, who were standing around, witnessing all that was going on.

CASE NUMBER 24

I will describe another uncommon problem that I came across while working in the Twin-Cities area of Minnesota, where I worked for a few years after I left the Dells Clinic at the end of 2002.

A middle-aged lady presented to me for the first time complaining of a number of nonspecific symptoms that she had been experiencing for some time. She complained of fatigue, occasional chills, mild headache, some joint aches and pains and feeling a bit dizzy at times. She also complained of intermittent fever. She denied having had any skin rashes. Her physical exam was not very revealing as to etiology of her complaints.

She had consulted a couple of providers in the recent past without a specific cause being found, and the treatment given being ineffective. I obtained a few blood studies, including a CBC (complete blood count). On this, I noted a significant thrombocytopenia (low platelet count), and a significant anemia.

As the season was summer, I had been thinking of Lyme disease at the time, although the patient had given no history of any tick bites. On seeing these results, however, I started thinking of Babesiosis, also a tick-borne infection. The same species of ticks that spread Lyme disease may also carry this. This disease is caused by a parasitic protozoa, which infests red blood cells, causing them to undergo hemolysis (break up), which causes a so-called "hemolytic anemia." Thrombocytopenia (low platelet count) is commonly present. The disease can be more severe in the immunocompromised, in the elderly, and in those who have no functioning spleen.

I then obtained tests specific for the diagnosis of Babesiosis and indeed, they confirmed this diagnosis. I was just "filling in" for a limited time at the clinic in which I was working, so I contacted an Infectious Disease specialist and referred the patient for treatment. The disease is treated with a Malaria-type drug. I did see her a couple of times soon thereafter. She improved very quickly, her symptoms abated, and her blood count was returning to normal. Babesiosis is a somewhat uncommon disease. Actually, I had been looking for this condition for some time, but this was the first case that I found.

CASE NUMBER 25

One afternoon, while seeing my schedule at the Dells Clinic, I received a call from a patient of mine who had just returned to his home. He had been working at his job in Madison, about fifty miles away, and had started feeling dizzy and left his job to drive home. On the phone, he told me of feeling so weak and dizzy at times, that he actually had to pull off on the shoulder of the road for a bit. Then, as he was talking, the phone line suddenly went silent. I couldn't get a response.

I knew where he lived in the bordering town of Lake Delton, so I got into my car and drove to his home. I found that he had passed out but was now responding. He was home alone as his wife was a school teacher and was away during the day. I called the ambulance and hospitalized him.

A workup revealed retroperitoneal bleeding from an arteriovenous malformation in the area of the kidney. He was then cared for in Madison, where surgery was performed, correcting his problem.

A few years later, the same patient came to the clinic one afternoon saying he had passed out in the shower at home, hitting his head. He complained of a bad headache. His sensorium was a bit compromised also, but he was essentially rational. After further discussion and with concerning findings of nuchal rigidity (stiff neck) on a physical exam, I became concerned that a subarachnoid hemorrhage had been responsible for his fall and his headache. Consequently, I immediately hospitalized him where a spinal tap revealed blood in the spinal fluid. He, indeed, had suffered a sub-arachnoid hemorrhage. I immediately called one of the neurosurgeons in Madison that I knew, discussed the situation with him, and transferred the patient there. He underwent surgery.

The surgeon told me later that he was very concerned during the surgery that the patient might not survive. He did, however—and made a full recovery.

CASE NUMBER 26

I'll end with a bit of humor...

As a matter of course, when one of my obstetrical patients went into labor and was hospitalized, I was usually at their bedside monitoring their situation and progress during labor. These were the days before fetal monitoring, routinely used today. Fetal heart tones, cervical dilation, mother's vital signs, etc., were serially checked. In this particular instance, the labor ceased to progress in an acceptable manner and a caesarian section delivery was indicated.

The patient's husband was not at the hospital at this time, and I wished to contact him as to our plans for the delivery. They lived in the countryside as they were farmers. I phoned their home but got no answer. Then, the mother-to-be, gave me the number of a neighbor who she thought could perhaps get word to her husband. I called there and a gentleman answered. I said that I was trying to get word to the patient's husband to tell him we were going to have to do surgery to deliver the baby, and I wanted him to know. Right away he responded, "Well, I could have told you that. She was as big as a house."

I thought, "Maybe I'll add his name to my list of Obstetrical consultants to contact when I have a problem with my OB patients."

MORE THOUGHTS

Since I began medical practice in the Dells in 1960, there have been remarkable advances in several modalities, both diagnostic and therapeutic, for so many medical issues. Listing all these would be a difficult, if not impossible, task. So many of them dramatically influenced my medical practice in so many areas. I will comment in some detail on a few of these.

THE TREATMENT OF ACUTE MYOCARDIAL INFARCTION (HEART ATTACK)

Several years after CPR and Defibrillation treatment of cardiac arrest became known, it was discovered that the final event that led to a heart attack was the rupturing of a coronary artery plaque, which led to the formation of a blood clot in that area which blocked the artery. Consequently, the cardiac muscle in the area downstream from this obstruction would not receive any blood flow, and this caused the symptoms of chest pain, etc. Unless this obstruction could be relieved, and quickly, the cardiac muscle downstream would not survive.

Subsequently, with this knowledge of an obstructing blood clot, thrombolytics—so-called "clot-busting drugs"—were developed. These became available and were administered intravenously and were about 65- to 70-percent successful in lysing the clot and reestablishing blood flow (opening the obstructed coronary artery). However, they needed to be given within a certain, limited time for best results. If the artery was opened, muscle damage to the heart could be limited. I was able to use these drugs many times.

Then, even later, PCI (percutaneous coronary intervention) was developed and soon became the standard of care of acute heart attacks. This procedure, in brief, involves taking the patient to the cardiac cath lab as soon as possible after a diagnosis of heart attack, inserting a catheter into the heart through a peripheral artery, injecting dye and taking a picture to determine the site of the obstruction in the artery. Then, another catheter device is inserted, the artery is expanded by inflating a balloon device and a metal stent is inserted in the area to keep the artery open. This had a higher rate of success, compared to the "clot-busting" drugs.

Again, however, the benefit of this procedure also depended on how quickly this could be done after the onset of symptoms. Another limit to this was the fact that many patients did not have access to a hospital with a cath lab within an appropriate time.

Both of the above procedures have had a positive impact on mortality from, and decreased the extent of damage to the cardiac muscle caused by, heart attacks.

THE TREATMENT OF PEPTIC ULCER

I will also offer a few comments on another problem that was fairly common in my early years of practice at the Dells Clinic: peptic ulcer—either duodenal or stomach, more commonly the former.

These patients were usually fairly symptomatic (abdominal pain between meals, etc.), and available treatment was really of quite minimal help. Treatment was usually by certain dietary restrictions, and the use of antacids, such as Amphojel, Gelusil and later, Maalox. Patients sometimes took Tums, Rolaids (calcium carbonate), even sodium bicarbonate, which gave fast, but not long-lasting, relief of symptoms. All of these medications worked by neutralizing stomach acid and raised the gastric pH.

I frequently saw complications of the ulcers, most commonly bleeding. Blood loss was often severe. No medical therapy of any significant value in stopping the bleeding was available. These patients would present with a history of black, tarry, foul-smelling, loose stools, which was due to passage of partially digested blood through the GI tract. Depending on the rapidity and length of time of the bleed, these patients sometimes presented with symptoms of blood-loss shock. They were admitted to the hospital, where blood transfusions were given.

Not uncommonly, the bleeding persisted, and after the administration of several units of blood, with bleeding showing no signs of subsiding, the patient was taken to surgery to control the bleeding. I assisted in several of these cases, and more than once I observed an ulcer crater with a blood vessel in the base, actively bleeding.

Perforation was another complication. I saw a few cases of this, where an ulcer over time would get deep enough to perforate the wall of the stomach or duodenum. Then the contents of air and gastric juices would flow freely out into the abdominal cavity. This resulted in severe pain. Exam would reveal a rock-hard abdomen on palpation, and the patient would not want to move. Plain abdominal x-rays would show evidence of free air in the abdominal cavity. These cases were a surgical emergency.

As time passed, there were significant advances made in the treatment of peptic ulcer. Two things revolutionized the treatment to a degree that today, one almost never encounters the above complications of serious bleeding or perforation.

The first was the development of new types of medications that worked not by *neutralizing* stomach acid, but by decreasing acid *production* by the stomach. First, so-called Histamine type 2 blockers, so called H2 blockers (e.g. Tagamet, Zantac, Pepcid) and somewhat later the more effective PPIs (proton pump inhibitors; e.g. Prilosec, Prevacid, Protonix, Nexium and others). These PPIs could actually heal an active ulcer in a matter of a few weeks. They could also be used to help prevent ulcers from forming in high-risk situations. They were also effective in other upper GI problems (e.g. Gastroesophageal reflux).

Secondly, a bacteria called Helicobacter Pylori was discovered to be the cause of most duodenal ulcers, gastric ulcers and gastric cancer. This was discovered by two

Australian physicians in the 1980's. In fact, they were rewarded with the Nobel Prize. This bacteria can be found in the wall of the stomach in many people. The presence of Helicobacter Pylori can be readily detected by relatively simple tests, and it can be eradicated, in the great majority of cases, by brief treatment with readily available and well-tolerated medications.

After the discovery of Helicobacter Pylori, and the PPI drugs, I never saw another severe GI bleed from ulcer disease. Additionally, gastric cancer has become relatively uncommon in the Western world.

THE TREATMENT OF CHRONIC HEPATITIS C

Another remarkable advance, just in 2014, is a new treatment for chronic Hepatitis C. Presently (2015), Hepatitis C is the leading reason for liver transplantation in the United States.

Hepatitis C is viral infection of the liver and is much more likely than Hepatitis B to go into a chronic stage after acute infection. Over the years, this may lead to cirrhosis, hepato-cellular liver cancer and liver failure. These complications often meant the need for liver transplantation.

Until now, drug treatment of Hepatitis C had been only moderately effective, as well as being associated with significant side effects. Last year, however, drugs—taken orally, and well tolerated—have been developed that will cure almost 100% of Hepatitis C. Although very expensive, so also is liver transplantation.

In addition to these three, more detailed examples, other areas of major improvement in treatment of so many chronic conditions occurred during my years of practice at the Dells Clinic. Of these, I will not comment in detail, but I feel they merit a mention.

There have been...

- new diagnostic radiographic modalities, such as Ultrasonography, CT scans, MRIs, PET scans, etc.

- major advances in therapeutic agents in every area of medicine: Infectious disease (multiple new antibiotics), Cardiovascular, Gastroenterology, Genitourinary, OB/Gynecology, Endocrinology, Neurology, Musculoskeletal, Dermatology, Psychiatry, Chemotherapy, etc.

- multiple new and better agents for treatment of Diabetes, Hypertension, Congestive Heart Failure, Asthma, Cancer and so many more conditions.

Take the treatment of Congestive Heart Failure, for example. When I started practice, Mercuhydrin injections, an organic-mercurial was commonly used as a diuretic in the treatment of Congestive Heart Failure along with Digitalis. Later, the thiazide diuretics became available and had some benefit when taken orally. It was several years later, however, that the loop diuretics such as furosemide (Lasix) became available, and this constituted a major advance in the area of diuretics in the treatment of heart failure. Even later, drugs in other categories further improved—and markedly so—the treatment of Congestive Heart Failure. I am referring to drugs such as Angiotensin Converting Enzyme Inhibitors, Beta-Blockers and Aldosterone Antagonists.

- new vaccines, very safe and effective, made available for Polio, Measles, Mumps, German Measles, Chicken Pox, Pneumococcal Pneumonia, Meningococcal and Haemophilus Meningitis, Hepatitis A, Hepatitis B, Herpes Zoster, Adult Pertussis, Rotavirus, Human Papilloma Virus, as well as improved Influenza and Rabies vaccines.

Pediatric Diphtheria, Pertussis and Tetanus vaccine (DPT), and the injectable Polio vaccine (Salk vaccine) were available when I started practice, as well as the Smallpox vaccine, which is no longer indicated or given in the United States.

- major advances in Radiotherapy, including Interventions by Interventional Radiologists, such as Ultrasound and CT guided biopsies, draining of internal abscesses, thoracocentesis, paracentesis, administration of chemotherapeutic agents to tumors, and much more.

- major advances in Cardiologist interventional procedures, such as Cardiac catheterization for many purposes, Angioplasty for heart attacks, Ablative treatment of arrhythmias, insertion of Pacemakers and Internal Defibrillators and other monitoring, diagnostic and treatment procedures.

- major advances in all types of surgery, such as Laparoscopic procedures and Robotic procedures.

- advances in Genetic and Molecular Biological knowledge which has led, among other things, to a whole new class of therapeutic agents, agents that modified the natural course of diseases, for example, DMARDS (disease-modifying, antirheumatic drugs).

- many new Diagnostic and Screening Tests, too numerous to count. One of particular note is the ability to check blood for Hepatitis B, Hepatitis C and HIV/Aids, making Blood transfusions so much safer.

All the above affected my practice tremendously in many ways. For example, almost all the "childhood diseases," once so common and affecting almost everyone without fail, are rarely seen anymore, due to the development of vaccines.

The advances noted above have resulted in PREVENTING DISEASE from ever occurring, through vaccines and screening tests, and if disease did occur, much improved DIAGNOSTIC ABILITY and much IMPROVED TREATMENT, resulting in much IMPROVED OUTCOME.

Bearing in mind these remarkable advances and results there is, however, one thing that bothers me, and I can support this concern to a certain degree by personal observation, having worked alongside so many Primary Care Physicians in my career. It is my perception that more recently trained physicians do not seem to have the expertise in doing, nor the diagnostic acumen gained from doing, a detailed, comprehensive history and physical exam, compared to those trained in my era. Instead, there seems to be a tendency to move quickly to getting "tests" of all types. Many times, I agree, tests are necessary and indicated, and we would be severely handicapped without them, but sometimes they can be superfluous, and at no small cost.

Admittedly, I am not privy to the details of today's training of primary care physicians. However, I wonder how comprehensive their training is before entering practice, given the scope of practice expected of primary care physicians these days. For example, many, if not most, of today's Family Practice physicians do not deliver babies, attend hospitalized patients, care for fractures or most trauma, including repairing lacerations (unless very simple), etc. Also, I suspect they are not expected to routinely provide even the initial care of most emergencies, such as heart attacks, diabetic complications, stroke and other common emergent situations. I realize this may be appropriate in most instances, but in certain situations there is, even today, a need for some degree of expertise in a broad range of emergent situations, especially in more rural areas.

Given the fact that the scope of practice of Family Practice primary care physicians is being encroached upon by the increasing numbers of Clinical Nurse Practitioners and Physician Assistants on one end and Sub-Specialists on the other, I wonder what special niche, if any at all, is left for Family Practitioners to fill. What, if anything, really separates them from alternative health care providers?

Furthermore, the burden of the rules and regulations of the Federal Government and Managed Care Organizations have not enhanced the attraction of entering the Family Practice environment—certainly not the type of practice that would be attractive to me, if I was entering the medical profession today.

In conclusion, I feel the ideal situation would be to have Primary Care Physicians undergo more comprehensive training to broaden their scope of practice, or at least be able to respond in an appropriate fashion to so many situations that they may come across in their practice. They would have at their disposal the current wide array of the multitude of advances discussed earlier. They would be better equipped to provide significant beneficial care to a wide range of problems. And still, when needed, they would have the readily available sub-specialized help, with rapid and safe transport.

A FINAL OPINION

The phenomenon of Managed Care "taking over" private practices and virtually eliminating physician involvement in decision-making, has, in my opinion, essentially destroyed the physician-patient relationship, which was so respected and treasured in past years by patients and doctors alike. This has happened to the extent that I now view Medicine as no longer a profession, but a business. Despite the sometimes flowery language in Managed Care's mission statements concerning quality and patient-centered care, I feel their top priorities too often lie elsewhere, and I feel most patients who have to deal with "today's system," will readily agree.

AGAIN, I WILL BE FOREVER THANKFUL FOR, AND GRATEFUL TO, ALL WHO CONTRIBUTED TO MY TRAINING IN PREPARING ME FOR THE PRACTICE I WAS TO ENCOUNTER IN MY CAREER AS A PRIMARY CARE PHYSICIAN

IN MY EARLY YEARS OF PRACTICE, OFTEN I WAS "911"

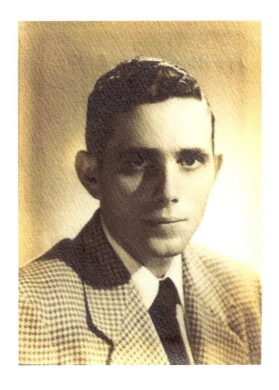

**GRADUATION
BUTLER UNIVERSITY
COLLEGE OF PHARMACY
1952
DEGREE – BS IN PHARMACY**

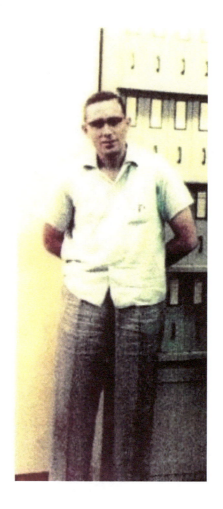

**NIGHT PHARMACIST
UNIVERSITY OF ILLINOIS
RESEARCH HOSPITAL
CHICAGO, ILLINOIS
1955-1959**

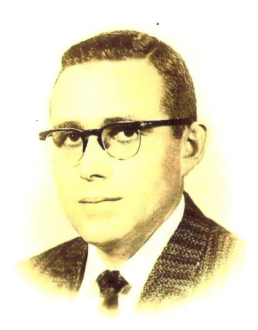

ADMITTED INTO MEMBERSHIP 1957

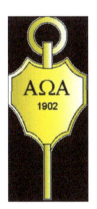

The **Alpha Omega Alpha Medical Honor Society**, commonly called **Alpha Omega Alpha** (**AΩA** or **AOA**), is a national honor society for medical students, residents, scientists, and physicians in the United States and Canada. Membership into AOA is one of the highest honors a student is eligible for during his or her four years of medical school, as only a small fraction of a class is even eligible for this distinction.

(*source: Wikipedia*)

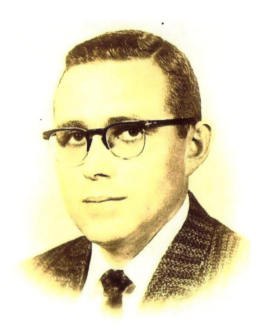

**GRADUATION
UNIVERSITY OF ILLINOIS
COLLEGE OF MEDICINE
NAVY PIER
CHICAGO, ILLINOIS
1959
DEGREE – DOCTOR OF MEDICINE**

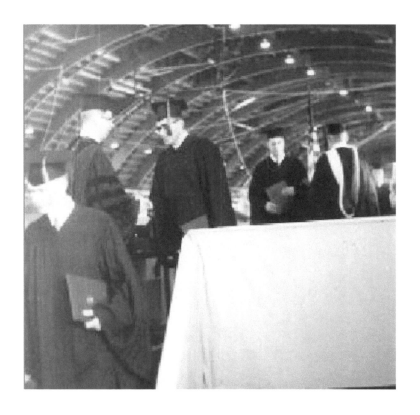

**GRADUATION
UNIVERSITY OF ILLINOIS
COLLEGE OF MEDICINE
NAVY PIER
CHICAGO, ILLINOIS
1959
DEGREE – DOCTOR OF MEDICINE**

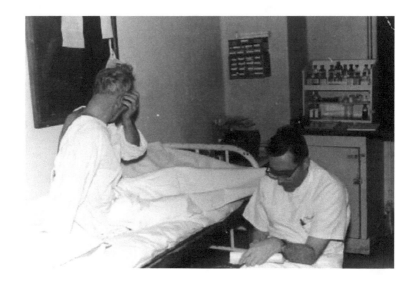

**HAROLD CONLEY MD
INTERN
COOK COUNTY HOSPITAL
CHICAGO, ILLINOIS
1959-1960**

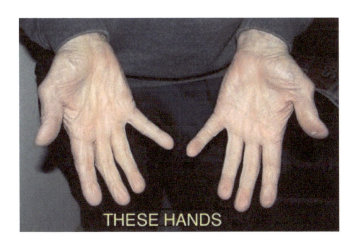

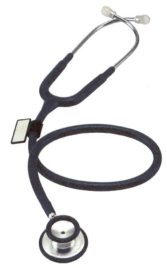

"TOOLS OF THE TRADE"
CIRCA 1960

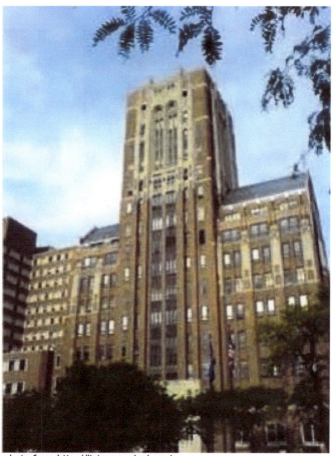

photo from http://livingnewdeal.org/

**UNIVERSITY OF ILLINOIS
COLLEGE OF MEDICINE
& RESEARCH HOSPITAL
CHICAGO, ILLINOIS
1955-1959**

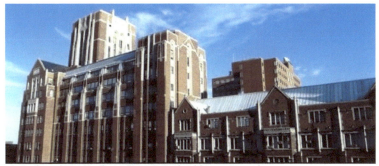
photo from http://collegeuniversitytoday.blogspot.com/

UNIVERSITY OF ILLINOIS COLLEGE OF MEDICINE & RESEARCH HOSPITAL CHICAGO, ILLINOIS 1955-1959

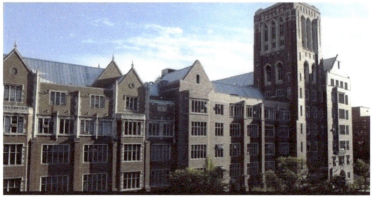
photo from http://chicago.medicine.uic.edu/

UNIVERSITY OF ILLINOIS COLLEGE OF MEDICINE CHICAGO, ILLINOIS 1955-1959

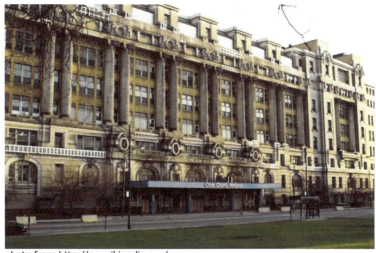
photo from http://en.wikipedia.org/

COOK COUNTY HOSPITAL
CHICAGO, ILLINOIS
INTERN
1959-1960

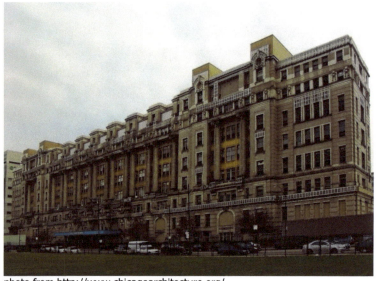
photo from http://www.chicagoarchitecture.org/

**COOK COUNTY HOSPITAL
CHICAGO, ILLINOIS
INTERN
1959-1960**

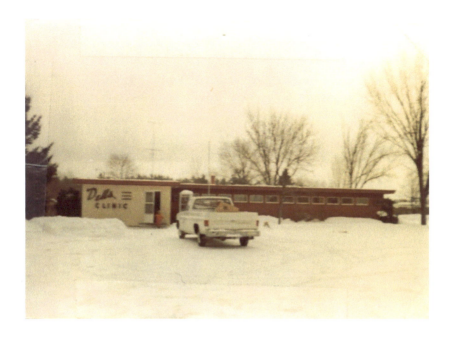

**DELLS CLINIC
WISCONSIN DELLS, WISCONSIN
1960 & BEYOND**

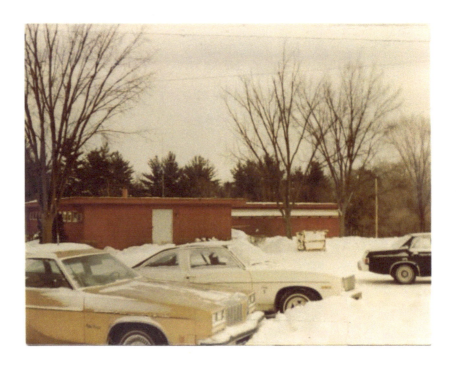

**DELLS CLINIC
WISCONSIN DELLS, WISCONSIN
1960 & BEYOND**

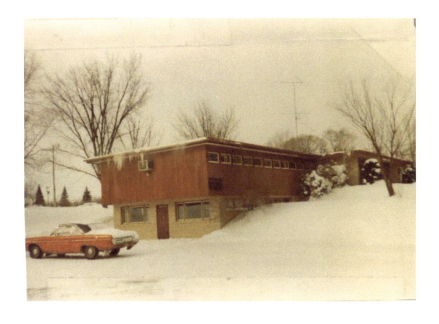

DELLS CLINIC
WISCONSIN DELLS, WISCONSIN
1960 & BEYOND

CPSIA information can be obtained
at www.ICGtesting.com
Printed in the USA
LVHW071234280719
625626LV00017B/787/P